THE PLEASANT SURPRISE

OF SOBRIETY:

figuring out your

recuperating interaction

By

Debbie H. Byrd

Copy right law (Debbie H. Byrd),2023

Table of content

Table of content

Introduction

Chapter 1

figuring out how to be level-headed

What Is Collectedness?

Step-by-step instructions to Remain Sober

6 Triggers of Backslide and How to Stay away from Them

The most effective method to Make Your Wellbeing Objectives S.M.A.R.T.

What are the 12 stages from a collectedness point of view?

Chapter 2

Being More Pleasant

Step-by-step instructions to Turn into a More Pleasant Individual

Chapter 3

nature and how to party sober

Ideas to remember as you venture outside

5 stages that can assist you with remaining focused

Chapter 4

mingling sober

Ways of Expressing No to Liquor When You Would rather not Drink

Creating Solid Connections in Recuperation

Chapter 5

dating and sex

Know about Co-dependency

Chapter 6

10 sober exercises for enslavement recuperation

Conclusion

Introduction

Ever sworn off alcohol for a month and found yourself drinking by the 7th? Think there's 'no point' in just one drink? Welcome! There are millions of us. 64% of Brits want to drink less.

Debbie H. Byrd was stuck in a hellish whirligig of Drink, Make horrible decisions, Hangover, Repeat. She had her fair share of 'drunk tank' jail cells and topless-in-a-hot-tub misadventures. But this book goes beyond the binges and blackouts to deep-dive into uncharted territory:

What happens after you quit drinking? This gripping, heart-breaking and witty book takes us down the rabbit-hole of an alternative reality. A life with zero hangovers, through sober weddings, sex, Christmases and breakups.

The pleasant surprise of sobriety, Debbie H. Byrd shines a light on society's drink-pushing and talks to top neuroscientists and psychologists about why we drink, delving into the science behind what it does to our brains and bodies. Much more than a tale from the netherworld of addicted drinking, this book is about the escape, and why a sober life can be more intoxicating than you ever imagined.

Whether you're a hopelessly devoted drinker, merely sober-curious, or you've already ditched the drink, you will love this book.

Chapter 1

figuring out how to be level-headed

What Is Collectedness?

Collectedness implies not being affected by a substance. Be that as it may, the word is much of the time utilized in various ways in various settings. Numerous 12-step programs recommend that collectedness implies complete forbearance — at absolutely no point in the future utilizing the substance.

Different definitions, notwithstanding, frequently centre around the course of recuperation and creating strategies for dealing with especially difficult times and propensities that help well-being and health over the long haul.

Complete forbearance might be the objective, however, actually, difficulties are normal.

It is assessed that up to 80% of the individuals who find long haul collectedness had somewhere around one backslide route.

Certain individuals experience numerous difficulties before they track down enduring recuperation. Your expectations might be great, however, it takes more than self-discipline to try not to have backslide.

There are different apparatuses accessible that can uphold your way to collectedness. Research recommends that while 12-step bunches are successful, individuals frequently don't proceed with their contribution at advantageous levels over the long haul.

One investigation discovered that common care groups can be pretty much as compelling as 12-step programs and may assist with working on the chances of progress for individuals who are focused on keeping a long period of complete restraint.

Step-by-step instructions to Remain Sober

Some say the best guidance for rookies to recuperate on the most proficient method to remain sober is straightforward: "Don't drink or utilize and go to gatherings." On the off chance that equation works for you, do it.

In any case, for a great many people, remaining sober isn't simply direct. The more methodologies you figure out how to distinguish triggers, adapt to pressure, and deal with your new level-headed life, the simpler it is to forestall backslide.

Distinguish Your Triggers

A major piece of forestalling backslide is figuring out your outside triggers, or individuals, spots, things, and circumstances that inspire considerations or desires related to substance use, as well as your interior triggers like sentiments, contemplations, or feelings related to substance use.

When you distinguish your greatest dangers, you can arrange to get ready for or keep away from them. A few normal triggers might include:

Stress

Close-to-home trouble

Ecological signals

Individuals who are as yet utilizing medications or drinking

Relationship inconveniences

Work or monetary issues

6 Triggers of Backslide and How to Stay away from Them

Perceive Backslide Cautioning Signs

A backslide can surprise you, for the most part since you don't perceive the admonition signs. A backslide starts sometime before you get a beverage or a medication and includes three stages: close-to-home backslide, mental backslide, and actual backslide.

Cautioning indications of backsliding include:

Getting back to habit-forming speculation designs

Participating in enthusiastic, pointless ways of behaving

Searching out circumstances affecting individuals who use liquor and medications:

Thinking less judiciously and acting less dependably

Winding up in a circumstance in which medication or liquor use appears to be a legitimate departure from the torment

Cautioning Indications of a Liquor or Medication Backslide

Get ready for PAWS

Post-intense withdrawal condition (PAWS) includes encountering withdrawal side effects that persevere past the detox period. Such side effects are much of the time connected with the state of mind and may incorporate peevishness, nervousness, discouragement, exhaustion, and rest issues.

Contingent upon the kind of reliance, PAWS can endure from a half year to two years after you quit utilizing medications or liquor.

The side effects engaged with PAWS can be an obstruction to recuperation if you don't watch out. As well as having the option to remember them, it's essential to know when to look for help.

On the off chance that PAWS is extreme or on the other hand on the off chance that you're encountering delayed side effects, a clinical expert can assist you with managing them and staying in recuperation without backsliding.

Keep away from Old Schedules and Propensities

It makes sense that assuming you quit your medication of decision however go on with your equivalent everyday practice, sticking around similar individuals and spots, and not rolling out any improvements in your conditions, slipping once again into your old ways of behaving and habits will be a lot more straightforward.

A portion of the prompt changes you should cause will be self-evident — like not staying nearby individuals that you utilized with or got drugs from. All things considered, you can't stick around your street pharmacist or old drinking amigos and hope to stay sober for extremely long.

You may likewise have to change your course to work or home to stay away from any triggers, individuals, spots, or things that make you need to utilize medications or drink once more.

Construct Solid Connections

Now that you are level-headed, you might have found that a portion of your past connections was undesirable as well as tremendously poisonous. It's not only your drinking mates and street pharmacists who can cause you problems — some of the time the individuals who are nearest to you can add to a backslide.

For instance, you might have fostered a mutually dependent relationship, or a relative, companion, or business might have been empowering you without knowing it.

That's what research shows assuming you keep up with these kinds of poisonous connections, your possibilities of backsliding are greater. To stay away from backsliding and stay sober, creating sound relationships is significant.

Get Backing

On the off chance that you find it challenging to make new, sober companions, take a stab at joining a care group. Investing more energy with strong friends and family and arranging exercises for the whole family can likewise assist you with fostering a better way of life and staying away from circumstances in which you would regularly drink or use drugs.

Looking for help from a therapist is likewise significant. A psychological well-being proficiency can assist you with adapting to a portion of the provokes you'll look on your way to collectedness.

A specialist can assist you with mastering new adapting abilities, foster new reasoning examples, and address any co-happening psychological well-being conditions that might make recuperation more troublesome.

Foster an Organized Timetable

Having a tumultuous or disarranged way of life can likewise frustrate your recuperation. Fostering an organized day-to-day and week-after-week timetable and sticking to it is significant.

An organized routine will assist you with accomplishing different objectives in your day-to-day existence, whether they are present moment (like being on time for work) or long haul (like returning to school and evolving professions).

Remaining sober is a high need, however, creating and seeking different objectives can assist you with keeping up with that collectedness.

The most effective method to Make Your Wellbeing Objectives S.M.A.R.T.

Practice Solid Living

Persistently abusing drugs or potentially alcohol can negatively affect your physical and close-to-home well-being, and now that you're in recovery, you'll need to focus on taking care of yourself and guaranteeing you have the determination to stay sober. Keys to a solid way of life include:

Practicing consistently

Setting aside a few minutes for sporting exercises and side interests

Eating customary, even dinners

Getting more than adequate, great-quality rest

Rehearsing unwinding methodologies, similar to care contemplation and yoga exercise can assist with keeping away from an enslavement backslide

Centre around Your Funds

Individuals in recuperation from a substance use jumble as often as possible have issues meeting business-related liabilities, keeping up with work, and overseeing cash. On the off chance that you were dynamic in your enslavement for a while, you might have created monetary issues.

Monetary difficulties and issues finding and saving businesses are significant triggers for backsliding; however, it is feasible to make baby steps and set your funds up. Simply remember that your enhancements will not come about by accident more or less.

Consider connecting with a professional restoration instructor or vocation mentor to assist you with refreshing your resume, practicing prospective employee meeting abilities, and finding occupations that match your abilities and experience.

When you accomplish a return to work, it's essential to make a financial plan and do whatever it may take to protect yourself as work pressure can be a backslide trigger.

Dealing with Your Cash Can Help Your Recuperation

Remain Cool and Quiet

Many individuals who abuse liquor or medications experience difficulty managing outrage. Whenever left uncontrolled, outrage can adversely affect your well-being and your enduring collectedness.

Outrage is an ordinary and regular inclination, yet how you manage it will affect keeping up with your recovery.

For some individuals with a substance use jumble, it's only a question of never having taken properly to oversee outrage. Converse with your specialist, other medical services supplier, or support about how to manage your displeasure in a manner that won't make you hurt yourself or others or go to liquor or medications.

Managing Outrage in a Solid Manner Is Significant

Manage Previous oversights: many people who advance into recuperation have left a ton of torment and experience afterward. Feeling remorseful or embarrassed about the past way of behaving or activities during dynamic enslavement is regular and sound.

Disgrace is having negative convictions about yourself and your self-esteem. Responsibility is having pessimistic sentiments about your past way of behaving. Individuals in recuperation can encounter a great deal of disgrace essentially for having become dependent in the first place.

On the off chance that these feelings become over the top, they can keep you away from recuperation. On the off chance that you are attempting to keep a level-headed way of life, those sentiments can become poisonous and add to backslide on the off chance that you don't manage them appropriately.

Most who find recuperation additionally find that they have sincerely harmed companions and friends and family and have many second thoughts about their past choices. To stay away from backsliding and remain sober, you genuinely should do whatever it may take to gain from your previous oversights and start to dependably carry on with life more.

Track down Equilibrium in Your Life

One normal misstep for individuals who are new to liquor and medication recuperation is subbing another enthusiastic way of behaving for their old one.8 Individuals new to recuperation can wind up moving toward their new eating regimen, practice program, work, and even cooperation in help bunches with an impulse that reverberations enslavement.

Although these new exercises are sound and useful, they can be a hindrance to enduring recuperation on the off chance that they become an exchange dependence to make up for the shortcoming left by the first enslavement. The mystery is to track down a good overall arrangement.

Discover that you have options and that you can keep up with control. On the off chance that any aspect of your life is crazy, it won't assist you with keeping up with enduring collectedness.

To Remain Sober, Stay away from Enthusiastic Ways of behaving

Observe Achievements

On the off chance that you're engaged with a 12-step program, you probably definitely know the significance of achievements. In these projects, it's standard to get plastic chips as you progress to the one-year point when you get a bronze coin.

Recognizing and commending the difficult work of recuperation is useful for keeping you propelled and reminding you why you moved toward collectedness in any case. Simply be certain that your prizes don't include medications or liquor. All things being equal, center around things, encounters, and exercises that will uphold your new, solid way of life.

Recommendation

Collectedness is an interaction and difficulties are normal. The most effective way forward for your recuperation from liquor or substance use is to consolidate a wide assortment of methodologies that will assist with encouraging achievement. Make sure to really focus on yourself, look for strong connections, and think about looking for help from a specialist.

What are the 12 stages from a collectedness point of view?

Conceding you are feeble over enslavement

Having confidence in a higher power

Giving up to a higher power

Taking an ethical stock

Conceding wrongs

Being prepared to have a more powerful eliminate your wrongs

Asking a higher power for help

Making a rundown of individuals you've violated

Offering to set things straight

Taking individual stock

Participating in supplication or contemplation

Rehearsing these standards and administration to the local area.

How long does collectedness exhaustion endure?

It relies upon what substance you are recuperating from, how long you've been utilizing it, and the amount you utilized. Collectedness exhaustion can last half a month to a couple of months. Be that as it may, in serious instances of post-intense withdrawal, side effects can endure as long as two years.

What is a collectedness date?

A collectedness date is a date that you quit utilizing a substance — for example, the day you quit drinking or quit utilizing drugs.

How would you compliment somebody on their collectedness?

Compliment somebody on their collectedness by communicating your help. You could say, "I'm truly pleased with you," or "I'm so glad to see you succeed." Try not to pose inquiries that are excessively private or zeroing in on the negative parts of their substance use.

What is viewed as long-haul collectedness?

Long haul collectedness is a general term — it implies various things to various individuals. In any case, many individuals believe long-haul collectedness to be moderation that has endured somewhere around one year.

Chapter 2

Being More Pleasant

Being pleasant to others is a significant method for spreading thoughtfulness and inspiration. As well as helping others, research recommends that this kind of prosocial conduct can likewise support your own psychological prosperity.

Step-by-step instructions to Turn into a More Pleasant Individual

Turning into a more pleasant individual isn't generally so hard as you would naturally suspect. There are things that you can do to show sympathy, compassion, and thoughtfulness in your ordinary collaborations with others.

Act with Thoughtfulness

Being a pleasant individual method of acting with thoughtfulness, and exploration recommends that consideration can emphatically influence your cerebrum. Individual thoughtful gestures trigger the arrival of oxytocin and endorphins and seem to cultivate the production of new brain associations.

Being benevolent is a self-building propensity. We hunger for the vibe and great impression of being kind, so one thoughtful gesture can without much of a stretch lead to another.

Try not to Be Excessively Basic

It very well may be difficult to be a pleasant individual when you're consumed by regrettable considerations. At the point when you wind up reprimanding somebody, attempt to embrace a more certain mentality. How might you re-evaluate what is happening and be more hopeful?

For example, on the off chance that a collaborator commits an error, stop before you scrutinize their work. Perhaps you view their misstep as a potential chance to help them as opposed to becoming irritated at them for not being awesome.

Tell The Truth

Remain consistent with yourself and your qualities. You can in any case communicate your thoughts pleasantly while telling the truth.

Being pleasant doesn't imply that you won't ever say "no" to individuals or that you do things that you would rather not do.

Defining solid and fair limits implies you're dealing with your psychological and close-to-home well-being. Being pleasant to others can come all the more naturally when you have a solid sense of reassurance and regard.

Be Pleasant to Yourself

The way that we treat ourselves, including our self-talk, assumes a significant part of the way we treat others. All things considered, how might we treat others pleasantly on the off chance that we don't treat ourselves pleasantly?

Notice how you converse with yourself and where you respond when something veers off-track — do you fault or rebuff yourself? Do you call yourself names? By rehearsing persistence and thoughtfulness toward ourselves, we make it more straightforward to be pleasant to other people.

Be Receptive

Life is brimming with change. At the point when we are going up against thoughts, circumstances, or individuals that are new to us, pessimistic feelings can emerge that make it challenging to be great.

Receptiveness is a fundamental quality for learning and engrossing data without judgment.4 Keeping a receptive outlook can assist you with exploring a new area while remaining mentally collected and loose.

It's a lot more straightforward to be pleasant when you're OK with yourself and your current circumstance — even in the midst of the many changes life tosses your direction.

Be Well mannered

Neighbourliness is just a single part of being great, however, it is a significant method for establishing and uplifting vibe in friendly collaborations.

Recollect that others' way of behaving doesn't have to cut yours down.

In the event that others are being unexpected or discourteous, answering with neighbourliness can be a method for redirecting the communication.

In ordinary discussions, straightforward words like "please" and "much obliged" can go quite far in showing somebody you value them.

Search for Ways of Being Useful

Really try to view little ways as accommodating in your day-to-day communications with others. From grinning at others in the supermarket to assisting a collaborator with an undertaking, being useful can be an extraordinary method for working on being pleasant over the course of your day.

Practice Absolution

Relinquishing past feelings of disdain and pardoning others can assist you with pushing ahead with a more inspirational perspective. It's more straightforward to be pleasant when you feel significantly better about others.

Pardoning yourself is likewise significant, so work on relinquishing negative encounters from an earlier time that keep you away from developing a more certain mentality.

Practice Appreciation

Put in almost no time every day contemplating something for which you are appreciative. You could find it supportive to keep an appreciation diary.

Research recommends that appreciation can have numerous medical advantages, including diminishing pressure and expanding satisfaction. Zeroing in on certain considerations can assist you with fostering a more uplifting perspective and can make it simpler to adapt to life's day-to-day problems and challenges.

Regard Others

Compassion and regard are additionally significant parts of delightfulness. During your day, attempt to see things according to the point of view of the others in your life and contemplate things that you can do to regard their requirements.

Regardless of whether you can't help contradicting what another person is doing, attempt to treat them with delightfulness and regard.

Regard individuals' experience also. On the off chance that you are meeting a companion, for example, attempt to arrive as expected and remain present during your discussions. Try not to gaze at your telephone excessively.

Practice undivided attention.

The specific meaning of "pleasant" can fluctuate starting with one individual and then onto the next. The field of character brain research recommends that there are at least one or two character characteristics related to this quality.

Therapists frequently portray the character with regard to five expansive aspects. One of these aspects is known as appropriateness. It incorporates a few characteristics that connect with how you treat others. For instance, a significant number of the qualities related to delightfulness, including thoughtfulness and compassion, are parts of pleasantness.

Research additionally recommends that appropriateness can then be separated into two fundamental parts: sympathy and respectfulness. Both of these characteristics assume a part in our thought process of "being great."

Sympathy is a characteristic that includes understanding and identifying with the close-to-home conditions of others and feeling moved to help.

Neighbourliness includes ways of behaving that are deferential to others and frequently persuaded by a longing for fairness.

Signs You're a Pleasant Individual

Individuals appear to appreciate your conversation.

You feel sympathy and compassion for other people.

You offer individuals certifiable commendations.

You pay attention to what others need to say.

You assume a sense of ownership with your slip-ups.

You're straightforward however deferential.

You're benevolent to other people.

You're thinking to yourself.

You're steady of others.

The Advantages of Being Great

Prosocial conduct is the term clinicians use to allude to activities worried about the prosperity, well-being, and sensations of others. At the end of the day, many "pleasant" ways of behaving like sharing, collaborating, and ameliorating are all prosocial activities that advance the government assistance of others.

Such ways of behaving clearly benefit those we help and encourage more noteworthy social connectedness. Notwithstanding, research additionally recommends that being pleasant to others can likewise help your own psychological well-being.

Expanded Engaging quality as an Expected Accomplice

Being a pleasant individual can make you more appealing as an accomplice. In a recent report distributed in the Diary of Character, members evaluated thoughtfulness as the absolute most significant trademark in a day-to-day existence partner. This implies individuals felt it was a higher priority than monetary possibilities, actual engaging quality, and a funny bone.

Better State of mind

Being pleasant feels significantly better. Research recommends that participating in kind and accommodating demonstrations can assist with working on your state of mind. In one review, specialists found that participating in thoughtfulness exercises every day for seven days expanded sensations of satisfaction and prosperity.

The investigation additionally discovered that the kinder demonstrations individuals played out, the more joyful they announced feeling. It additionally didn't make any difference on the off chance that these thoughtful gestures were coordinated toward companions, outsiders, or even oneself — all had a similarly certain effect.

Diminished Pressure

Delightfulness may likewise assume a part in pressure help. Studies recommend that being pleasant may likewise assist with peopling adapting all the more successfully to the impacts of pressure. For instance, in one review, specialists found that individuals who performed thoughtful gestures announced feeling less pressure and antagonism.

Expanded Thoughtfulness

Research has additionally demonstrated the way that thoughtfulness can be infectious. One investigation discovered that helpful ways of behaving will in general have an outpouring impact, spreading up to three levels of detachment from the source.

This implies that being pleasant to others is probably going to make them be good to others too, setting off an influx of kind and helpful ways of behaving inside interpersonal organizations.

Interesting points

While there are obviously a few significant advantages, being pleasant can likewise have a few disadvantages. This is especially obvious if they should be pleasant and obstructs certifiable correspondence and credibility.

A few possible pessimistic results of smothering your genuine sentiments with an end goal to be "pleasant" include:

Close-to-home explosions: On the off chance that you are continually subduing your actual contemplations and feelings only for introducing a "pleasant" persona, odds are those sentiments will ascend to the surface sooner or later. Tension might keep on working until some pressure sets off a response, which could appear as an unexpected explosion of peevishness or through and through outrage.

Sensations of disdain: Concealing your genuine sentiments or denying what you truly need since those feelings or wants are not viewed as "pleasant" can eventually prompt sensations of hatred or sharpness. This can make an explosive impact and adversely influence your associations with others.

Shallow connections: On the off chance that you're not expressing the things you truly need in a relationship for trying not to struggle and be great, it might imply that you're not uncovering your legitimate self to other people. This frequently brings about connections that need both profundity and closeness. There might be not many contentions and clashes, however, there is likewise an absence of association and closeness.

While shallow delightfulness can be a pessimistic power, that doesn't imply that you shouldn't endeavour to be a pleasant individual. The key is to zero in on attractiveness driven by thought and care and not by a counterfeit facade of respectfulness that covers your genuine sentiments.

Note

There are a lot of ways that you can integrate delightfulness into your day-to-day existence. You could begin by showing your appreciation for somebody in your life or chipping in for a purpose you care about. Being pleasant feels significantly better — making delightfulness a propensity is much of the time its own prize.

It's alright on the off chance that you're battling to be a more pleasant individual. Like any expertise, being a more pleasant individual might take time and exertion. On the off chance that you're battling, you might wish to address a specialist or prepare psychological well-being proficiently to deal with any obstructions.

Chapter 3

nature and how to party sober

Nature is extraordinarily gorgeous. Contingent upon where you reside, you may not invest a lot of energy appreciating or contemplating nature. Be that as it may, on the off chance that you battle with your psychological well-being, investing energy in nature might be exactly what you really want. You needn't bother to be an outside individual to appreciate all that nature brings to the table. Let loose a day and go out to a state park or a remote path. You wouldn't believe every one of the advantages you experience and appreciate. As you go on in your recuperation, you might see that your psychological well-being changes. Finding what gives you pleasure and solace ought to be viewed as one of your fundamental objectives. Now and again it can turn out to be not difficult to turn out to be so focused on your collectedness and your well-being that you neglect to have a good time. The battle that inclination and make sure to find satisfaction while you keep up with your collectedness and objectives.

Ideas to remember as you venture outside.

Dedicate Your Time

Dedicate some time when you head out into nature. We as a whole carry on with occupied existences, which can undoubtedly be energizing your psychological well-being battles. Free up as much time as possible and essentially loosen up in the regular environmental elements accessible to you. Do whatever it takes not to contemplate all of the work you need to do or undertakings you really want to achieve. Focus on yourself, and be aware of your environmental elements.

Zeroing in on your psychological prosperity is something you most likely buckled down on during treatment. You figured out the fact that committing uninterrupted alone time is so significant. Be that as it may, setting aside a few minutes for yourself can be trying to recollect as you progress once more into society. Our days are jam-stuffed, and we live in a general public that celebrates being occupied. Recollect what you endeavoured to accomplish and take your power back. On the off chance that you think of yourself as battling, connect for help. There is no disgrace in requiring support as you explore a level-headed way of life.

Notice the Little Things

While you are out in nature, attempt to see the little things. Set aside some margin to take a gander at every one of the wildflowers loosening up towards the sun or the little honey bees humming through the tall grass. We lead such tumultuous and relentless lives that we neglect to interrupt and see the magnificence surrounding us. At the point when we can see the magnificence around us, we can focus our psyches and view it as our internal quiet.

Finding our internal quiet is an incredible asset. Stress, nervousness, and triggers will be essential for our lives; they are unavoidable. Figuring out how to find your solidarity and ground yourself when they strike is fundamental. Figuring out how to do this can require some investment. Be that as it may, it is worth the effort, and you will express gratitude toward yourself for investing the energy when you wind up in an awkward circumstance.

Recognize Your Sentiments

As you are strolling through nature, get some margin to see how you feel. Do you contemplate anything specifically? Do you feel quiet? Show improvement over what you do during the ordinary, active seasons of life. Assuming being in nature assists you with managing the anxieties of life and finding your quiet, then, at that point, that can be useful to your psychological well-being. You may likewise see that being in nature assists you with handling feelings, thinking with an unmistakable psyche, and figuring out objectives. Driving a level-headed way of life is an exceptionally certain decision, however, it accompanies pressure, very much like all the other things throughout everyday life. Figure out how to deal with the pressure and track down your satisfaction.

Investigate Beyond Your Usual range of familiarity

Use your available energy in nature to investigate beyond your usual ranges of familiarity. Frequently we stay inside our usual range of familiarity in light of the fact that doing so is agreeable and it is protected. Step outside your zone and take a stab at a genuinely new thing. You will start to track down solace in your uneasiness.

You can encounter a mind-boggling thrill in attempting new exercises and investigating new spots. You might see that getting out of your usual range of familiarity can assist you with keeping up with your psychological well-being and generally speaking prosperity.

Investigate new spots, attempt new exercises, and connect in headings you never figured you would. You are a strong individual, and enslavement no longer controls you. End your life back and appreciate finding yourself once more. Enslavement consumed you, and you most likely failed to remember every one of the exercises you once delighted in. Partake in your life once more, each new movement in turn. Take your loved ones and investigate together. Investing energy in nature can help you in countless various ways, both with yourself and with those you love.

Investing energy in nature can be magnificent. Greenspace can assist with peopling work through injury, enslavement, or psychological well-being battles. We are one of a kind, and tracking down the right movement to assist your psyche and body with discovering a lasting sense of reconciliation is an extraordinary objective to have.

While you are in nature, attempt to contemplate your excursion to collectedness and all of the difficult work you have done. Dedicate an opportunity to interfacing with the nature around you while being aware of what you are feeling. Nature can assist us with seeing the little things and valuing our battles.

Around here at The Visitor House, we adopt an all-encompassing strategy for recuperation. We realize that everybody is on their own excursion and requires various degrees of help. Many individuals need to proceed with help even in the wake of accomplishing a level-headed way of life.

Step-by-step instructions to party sober

There's a famous misguided judgment about collectedness that the party closes when we quit drinking. In opposition to mainstream thinking, your life doesn't need to become exhausting, everyday practice, and unexciting when you get level-headed. Recuperation appears to be unique for everybody, except on the off chance that mingling is something you are enamoured with, you shouldn't need to surrender each party and night out in light of the fact that you never again drink. All in all, what do you do?

Contemplating celebrating sober can be overwhelming, however, following these:

5 stages that can assist you with remaining focused.

1. Track down a beneficial occasion to join in

Let's just get real for a moment, when I was drinking, I went to for the most part, every occasion, get-together, party, birthday festivity, wine night, or supper where beverages were being served. I never said no. I was searching for a party constantly. In collectedness, I chose to just go to occasions that are advantageous. What's the significance here? It implies that I just need to go to occasions that fill a need, celebrate somebody I care about, recognize a specific event, or encourage me. Try not to go too simple to follow through with something. It could cause you to feel awkward being around liquor and those circumstances.

2. Go with companions you have a solid sense of reassurance and are agreeable around

At the point when I was drinking, I additionally went out with everybody. I had a wide range of gatherings of companions and when I needed to follow through with something, I would go down the rundown and call everyone until somebody consented to spend time with me. I had companions who I never truly talked with separated from when we were drinking. They filled a need for me; I realized they would continuously be down to party.

In collectedness, I've come to understand that to live it up in a party setting, I really want to feel great around the companions I'm with. I don't ordinarily go out to party with arbitrary individuals any longer. I feel excessively defenceless and awkward. I appreciate going out with companions who know me.

They comprehend I don't drink and they are there for me on the off chance that I really want support during the evening.

Being a piece of a level-headed local area, similar to Recuperation Lift, meetup gatherings, or Facebook networks, can be an effective method for meeting companions who are comprehension of your circumstance.

3. Continuously have a departure course prepared

I generally give this tip to anybody recently level-headed, any clearheaded individual who adventures out to a get-together, and any individual who needs to know how to party securely and sober. A delightful aspect concerning collectedness is that you can continuously commute home following an evening out on the town. Assuming you have your own vehicle, drive yourself to the occasion you're going to so that when you need to leave, you can do as such without looking out for any other individual. On the off chance that you begin to feel awkward, you have the opportunity to leave immediately. You won't be guaranteed to require your own vehicle to do this, however, make certain to design another choice — whether that be a ride-share administration (like Uber or Lyft), a taxi, or heading back home. Make an arrangement ahead of time so that you will not need to sit around idly for any other individual. Your collectedness starts things out.

4. Get a beverage to hold

This is an individual inclination, however, I like to arrange a beverage to convey and taste. A few bars and clubs have non-fermented lager, however, on the off chance that this isn't your thing, you can continuously get water, pop, or some other scrumptious liquor-free cocktail. It's recognizable to me to hit the dance floor with a beverage in my grasp and presently it's a special reward that my beverage doesn't cause me to feel entertained or urge me to fall.

5. Have some good times!

This is maybe the main component of celebrating sober: Have some good times. On the off chance that celebrating sober appears to be too distressing or overpowering, perhaps it's simply not the perfect opportunity in your collectedness or the right occasion to join in. Gatherings and clubs may not be places you find agreeable any longer. Celebrating sober ought to encourage you, not terrible! There's no disgrace in saying you're not prepared to associate in a setting where liquor is available, or that you simply feel really awkward at specific spots with specific individuals. In collectedness, we need to figure out how to support ourselves. Safeguard your recuperation, your prosperity, and your very own solace levels.

Keep in mind, a definitive objective for living sober is to get back to a far superior life, liberated from the shackles of liquor and medications. What preferable method for doing that over to have a good time, not regardless of your collectedness, but rather as a result of your temperance. The pleasant I have today is not quite the same as the great I had when I drank in light of the fact that it accompanies a protected feeling of opportunity.

Chapter 4

mingling sober

 the inquiry everybody in collectedness poses to themselves:

Will my companions actually need to spend time with me on the off chance that I'm tasting Perrier rather than Laurent-Perrier?

It's insane, however, telling your group of friends you don't drink is some of the time harder than not savouring the primary spot. Collectedness is far beyond a choice about your actual well-being and close-to-home prosperity — it tremendously affects your public activity.

Try not to anticipate that everything should be something very similar

Your public activity is different now — however, that is something worth being thankful for. You're unique, as well. A tremendous defining moment for me was tolerating that this is no joking matter, and however much I should hide it away from plain view, I can't. It's tremendous. I used to self-sedate with quite possibly of the most habit-forming drug on the planet, and I don't do that any longer. I've gone from being one of the drunkest individuals at the party to being (every now and again) the main sober individual. Obviously, things will be unique.

Realize that time will fabricate certainty

Liquor used to be my familiar object in any friendly circumstance I felt restless or awkward on dates, family parties, evenings out with bunches of ladies, work blenders, and so forth. I met my life partner before I got level-headed so I've never needed to explore sober dating, however, its simple idea gives me the most horrendously terrible sort of goose bumps.

Close to the furthest limit of my drinking days, the apprehension about losing that familiar object was my fundamental justification for not stopping. I won't lie: I was restless and awkward a great deal at get-togethers at the beginning of collectedness, so I needed to carry on like everything was cool. I actually have a periodic midsection gripping second when I stroll into a party sober, however as my trust in my choice develops, they're rare.

Trust your companions to be there

Your genuine ones, in any event. Collectedness can fascinatingly affect companionships. A portion of my companions has required a brief period to conform to my critical life decision. That is cool with me. Two or three others have floated away with practically no injury on one or the other side — I suspect my collectedness may essentially have sped up an unavoidable developing separated process. My actual companions were there for me when I was dropping at parties and hurling toward the rear of taxicabs, and they're there for me now.

I'm likewise framing new companionships since I'm committing the time I used to spend drinking or nursing headaches to different things: yoga, swimming, composing, publishing content to a blog — what John Mendelson, a teacher at the College of California at San Francisco and clinical enslavement master, calls "another social existence where drinking isn't the main capability of the party."

"Previous consumers might have to look for and join this world," he says. "Supper, work parties, and any unequivocally liquor-related occasions can be a test to recently sober individuals so you really want an arrangement on the off chance that you will go to these."

Make a reinforcement arrangement

Mendelson has more guidance for making those off-kilter social events somewhat simpler: Take your own liquor-free beverages with you any place you go. I like to have pink lemonade or ginger lager on draft consistently — I keep a reserve in my vehicle since, indeed, I'm additionally now the assigned driver. Furthermore, perhaps take a level-headed companion with you for moral help. (Note: No one has your back like an individual sober sister or sibling.)

Preparing is significant, and on the off chance that a circumstance is probably going to be a high gamble, it's totally fine for the arrangement to just be to quit, says Imprint Willenbring, who drove the Division of Treatment and Recuperation Exploration at the Public Establishment on Liquor Misuse and Liquor addiction (NIAAA) from 2004 to 2009 and was answerable for supervising research on liquor use jumble at colleges around the US. Another way, every arrangement ought to incorporate a departure plan. "On the off chance that you're feeling all around enticed, promptly leave," he says. "There's no benefit to testing your self-discipline."

Have a reaction prepared to the drinking question

At a few focuses during early collectedness, you're most likely going to get inquired as to for what reason you're not drinking. Willenbring suggests having a speedy expression primed and ready.

for example, "I simply find I feel significantly improved on the off chance that I don't drink." Blast. "On the off chance that somebody is industrious, consider answering, 'Does my not drinking make you self-conscious?'" he adds. "Individuals under collectedness have found this line of request rapidly and deferentially." On the off chance that that doesn't work, or on the other hand, assuming you feel under tension from companions to drink, here you need to scrutinize those connections.

"For some individuals, collectedness is standard and there are practically zero disparagements of non-consumers," Mendelson says. "Individuals in these gatherings are companions since they have comparative work, sporting, and proficient interests.

On the off chance that your gathering is worked around drinking acquiring acknowledgment for conduct not rehearsed by the group can be hard. For individuals mulling over a level-headed way of life, they will probably have to foster new companion gatherings and exercises. They are there — you should simply track down them."

As a last resort, simply remain at home. Truly. Take as much time as necessary with this entire thing, and maintain the attention on yourself. In the initial not many long stretches of collectedness, when I was turning myself in tangles attempting to sort out some way to tell individuals I was done drinking, the main other sober individuals I realize IRL told me, "The main discussion you really want to have is with yourself." It's a very decent mantra for the recently level-headed.

Being level-headed doesn't need to mean surrendering your public activity, yet overseeing collectedness in a group environment (particularly when liquor is involved) can be somewhat of a test. You might have many worries about going out in the wake of stopping drinking.

Could I at any point have some good times without drinking?

How might my companions respond?

Will I feel reluctant without a little fluid mental fortitude?

Could I at any point say "no" and stick to it?

On the off chance that you're in early recuperation, you'll need to avoid what is happening where liquor or medications are involved for quite a while. These conditions can set off desires and put you in danger of relapse.

Assuming you have chosen to scale back liquor for your well-being, or you're more settled in your collectedness, social conditions that include drinking might be simpler to explore. All things considered, being ready and having an arrangement can assist you with getting a charge out of going out after you've stopped drinking.

Have a Legitimate Talk with Your Companions

It ultimately depends on you to choose how much data to share and who to impart it to. You unquestionably don't need to legitimize your choice. Certain individuals drink, and certain individuals don't. Everybody has their own decision to make, and not a glaringly obvious reason is required.

On the off chance that you have old buddies who are probably going to help your endeavours, you could choose to have an immediate and legitimate discussion with them. Let them know that you intend to keep away from liquor or that you're scaling back.

Tell them how they might help. Maybe you'd see the value in a level-headed mate, or another person remaining sober with you when you go out or assisting you with opposing the compulsion to drink. Or on the other hand, perhaps you'd, in any case, prefer to hang out together, however not in bars. You could try and still prefer to do exactly the same things — like playing a game of cards or watching motion pictures together — however without liquor.

Ideally, a portion of your companions will uphold your choice. As a matter of fact, some of them could likewise be contemplating scaling back their own liquor use and be enlivened by you.

Be Ready for Individuals' Responses

While a portion of your companions might be absolutely steady in your choice, others might appear to be uninterested or answer in a negative manner. Your collectedness could act as a wake-up call to your "drinking mates" that they're polishing off unfortunate measures of liquor, or work up a touch of nervousness on the off chance that they feel awkward mingling sober. Or on the other hand, they may essentially maintain that you should share close by them since they think you'll all have some good times together while drinking.

Simply realizing a couple of potential responses will assist with guaranteeing that you're not overwhelmed and you're ready to adapt:

Irritating: Your companions might make statements like, "Come on, can you if it's not too much trouble, simply have one beverage to relax a bit?"

Prodding: You might get ridiculed for being "exhausting" or "faltering." A few companions could say you can't deal with your liquor or that you're getting too old to even consider drinking.

Persuading: Your companions could attempt to go about like they're helping you out by getting you a beverage, so you can "have a great time." Or, they might attempt to persuade you that on the off chance that you simply have one beverage, they won't tell anybody.

Peer pressure: Your buddies could pick on you a piece and attempt to convince you to have a beverage. They might try and pass out a series of shots and attempt to demand that you participate.

Conflict: An irritated companion might try and stand up to you and demand that your reluctance to drink is an indication of something greater, similar to a "controlling accomplice" or "an emotional meltdown."

It's additionally essential to be ready for the drawn out transforms you could insight from your choice to stop drinking, including:

Being progressively transitioned away from social circumstances: You might get less friendly solicitations over the long run once your companions understand that your choice not to drink won't change.

Being marked a particular way: On the off chance that liquor assumes a significant part in your companions' lives, you could get named as the "level-headed companion" or the "wearing one out."

Being welcome to be the assigned driver: You could observe that you're possibly welcome on occasions when your companions anticipate that you should be their assigned driver.

An adjustment of your companionship elements doesn't need to be something terrible, be that as it may. You could find the shift inviting. There's consistently an opportunity that you'll appreciate discussions with your companions more when you're level-headed. Furthermore, you might try and find that they value you more or regard your choices.

What's more, regardless of whether your companionships change such that you could do without, don't surrender. You could possibly make another friend network or essentially choose to spend time with your old buddies in various areas and times when liquor isn't the fundamental concentration.

Go to Spots That Don't Serve Liquor

Quite possibly the most straightforward thing you can do to abstain from drinking — and to try not to need to account for yourself — is to go to places that don't serve liquor.

Bistros, cinemas, historical centres, libraries, and drive-through eateries are only a couple of spots that aren't probably going to serve cocktails. Search for places locally that are without liquor — from rancher's business sectors to neighbourhood theatres, you'll probably find a lot of spots that don't serve liquor.

You could go out alone as you start this new section of your life. Or on the other hand, you could welcome your companions to go along with you in these spots as a method for empowering sober exercises.

Foster a Couple of Go-To Reactions

Clearly, you're not liable to stay away from liquor constantly. Weddings, shows, and even craftsmanship exhibitions for the most part serve liquor. Furthermore, obviously, your companions might need to go to bars, clubs, or different occasions where liquor is one of the fundamental attractions.

To be more ready, it's essential to foster some venture out in front of time for how you'll considerately turn down a beverage or handle inquiries concerning for what reason you're not drinking.

Contingent upon your solace level and the individual asking, you could choose to offer an immediate, honest reaction. Here are a few choices:

"I chose to quit drinking for some time."

"I'm not keen on drinking this evening."

"I surrendered liquor."

"I'm scaling back my drinking."

"I won't drink for some time."

"I'm level-headed inquisitive."

"I'm driving this evening, so I'm not drinking."

"I enjoyed some time off from drinking, and I love the manner in which I feel now. So I don't want to begin again any time soon."

Obviously, you don't have to account for yourself. A straightforward, "I'm drinking seltzer this evening," is sufficient. In any case, on the off chance that you realize your companions are probably going to give you trouble, or you realize that you will run into individuals who will demand you drink, having a couple of canned reactions can keep you from being taken unsuspecting.

Ways of Expressing No to Liquor When You Would rather not Drink

Have a Non-Cocktail Close by

Having something in your grasp consistently is useful. So on the off chance that you go to a spot that serves liquor, perhaps you can promptly arrange a non-cocktail.

On the off chance that you go to somebody's home, bring your own beverage. Whether you have filtered water or a protein shake with you, keeping a beverage in your grasp can keep individuals from offering you liquor. It will likewise assist you with declining all the more effectively on the off chance that you are offered a beverage since you can say, "Not this time, I as of now have one."

Think Fun

At the point when you stroll into a circumstance accepting that you can't have some good times level-headed, this is probably going to be an unavoidable outcome. You could try and disconnect yourself or keep away from living it up — which will then, at that point, build up your conviction (and others) that being level-headed makes fun incomprehensible.

Go into the circumstance with an inspirational perspective, and make the best of your time, regardless of whether you're the only one not drinking. You could really find that being level-headed is more agreeable than you anticipated

Make a Leave Excuse

On the off chance that you go out with individuals who are drinking and you're not having a great time, or you're truly enticed to drink yourself, then, at that point, you'll need to early leave. This is particularly significant on the off chance that you're heading off to someplace where you used to continuously drink previously. The bar or a similar club you used to visit while drinking might be a trigger for you.

While you can simply leave or say what you need to do without offering a motivation behind why you could find it's more useful to have a prearranged excuse to escape what is happening rapidly. A couple of models:

You need to rise and shine ahead of schedule for an occasion.

You're not feeling completely ideal.

You have plans to meet another companion.

On the off chance that you're in recuperation and feel particularly delicate or are longing for liquor even after you leave the climate, make certain to look for help. Call a confided-in companion or relative or go to a gathering at a close by help bunch.

Plan a Useful Morning Later

You could observe that quite possibly of the most outstanding aspect of not drinking is that you don't die the following daytime resting and feeling hungover. So take full advantage of the time you gain by accomplishing something agreeable or useful.

Go for a run, clean the house, or get things done. Then, at that point, take the remainder of your day to partake in your time. Having additional significant investment could persuade you to keep going without liquor.

Attempt New Things with Your Companions

On the off chance that your companions are in the mood for attempting things that don't include liquor, you can make a few ideas.

Welcome them to go to a recreation area, a historical centre, or climbing.

Pursue a class or new movement together.

You could find that you get to realize each other much better while you're making new recollections — as opposed to waiting around in the standard, worn-out bars. They could have some good times investigating new spots and attempting new things with you.

Search Out Individuals Who Don't Drink

You might have to move your group of friends to incorporate individuals who don't drink. This might appear to be extreme from the outset. On the off chance that you're encircled by individuals who make liquor a major piece of their lives, it can feel like everybody drinks.

Be that as it may, as a general rule, there are a lot of individuals out there who don't drink — and who are searching for companions who don't drink. You simply need to track down them. You could attempt new exercises with the goal that you can meet sober individuals, including:

Join a worker association.

Go to occasions that don't serve liquor.

Join web-based entertainment bunches for individuals who take part in sober exercises.

At the point when you get along with such individuals, you'll probably find that they do a lot of exercises that don't include liquor — like climbing, skiing, messing around, or fishing. Furthermore, you could try and find that you appreciate doing these sorts of things substantially more than exercises that include liquor.

Creating Solid Connections in Recuperation

Gain from Your Encounters

Think about each level-headed outing of an investigation. You could commit a few errors — like drinking when you didn't expect to or contending with somebody who offers you a beverage. In any case, you additionally could find that you are more joyful when you're not drinking, or that you truly appreciate discussions with individuals more when you're level-headed.

Gain from each insight. The data you remove can assist you with keeping on making your best life.

Notwithstanding why you choose to change your drinking propensities, mingling sober can feel frightening. Assuming you observe that you're attempting to stay away from liquor, or you're feeling desolate and disconnected, think about looking for proficient assistance. A specialist can uphold your endeavours and assist you with finding the methodologies that turn out best for you, your well-being, and your life.

Chapter 5

dating and sex

Notwithstanding what your identity is, connections are brimming with challenges — dating a recuperating alcoholic accompanies its own arrangement of hardships. In spite of the fact that we have issues with diminishing somebody's relationship achievement in light of this particular reality about them, their recuperation process is a critical component in any case.

Cherishing somebody in recuperation can require additional comprehension and compassion, as well as persistence and energy. Monitoring your accomplice's recuperation interaction and supporting their collectedness is fundamental for an effective relationship.

Dating a recuperating alcoholic will require serious responsibility and commitment, very much like recuperation.

Concerns Well defined for Cherishing Somebody in Recuperation

Heartfelt connections of any sort are much of the time brimming with potential chances to dive more deeply into yourself and your friends and family. Circumstances that would shake a conventional relationship can hit ones where one or the two accomplices are in recuperation significantly harder. Coming into the relationship, put forth a valiant effort to understand what you're getting into by being taught issues well-defined for connections in recuperation. Assuming the two players are available to conversation about triggers and feelings, it will improve the probability that both the relationship and recuperation will go on emphatically.

What We See Ourselves Means for How We Act in a Relationship

An existence with an accomplice in dynamic enslavement or recuperation will frequently prompt numerous horrendous circumstances and close-to-home unpredictability. This tendency towards pressure — joined with a heartfelt connection's consistently fluctuating interests — can make a back-and-forth movement of having a decent outlook on ourselves.

Cherishing somebody in recuperation will require an uplifted consciousness of the impact you have on your accomplice and what the contention between you means for your own healthy identity.

Utilizing that mindfulness and abilities you have acquired, you can uphold your accomplice in recuperation while guaranteeing that you each put resources into self-advancement.

Dating a recuperating alcoholic or somebody in recuperation will require more unmistakable consolations and backing strategies. The degree of need clearly will fluctuate contingent upon the people and relationship.

Frequently those in recuperation have battled the vast majority of their existence with a mental self-portrait and self-esteem. Enslavement just intensifies these circumstances. For the most part, they convey a profoundly situated feeling of disgrace in what their identity is and what they have done.

Recuperation carries the potential chance to confront those previous injuries and re-establish a sound perspective on the self. An effective recuperation relies upon it.

While cherishing somebody in recuperation, the need to address these injuries ought to be fundamentally important in the mending system.

What's with this large number of Sentiments?

An ordinary individual on a typical day can encounter a downpour of feelings from beginning to end. An individual in recuperation is the same, with the exception of these feelings will generally be more extraordinary and faltering. While cherishing somebody in recuperation, it is important to get ready for this surge of fluctuating and extraordinary feelings. Recuperating from enslavement — particularly liquor dependence — incorporates recapturing the capacity to deal with one's own feelings without involving substances as a bolster or redirection.

Dating somebody in recuperation makes you a critical piece of their help group. During the most crucial times, give criticism to your accomplice about their appearance or feelings through conduct and activities. Inside these discussions is where they can turn around unfortunate behaviour patterns and layout sound ones.

A steady accomplice doesn't empower disastrous ways of behaving or permit disparaging self-talk. Considering your accomplice responsible for the manner in which they respond is basic.

Might You at any point Trust a Recuperating Alcoholic?

Everybody has a set degree of confidence in new connections. For the most part, this is semi-foreordained by previous encounters. While dating a recuperating alcoholic or somebody in recuperation, there's a decent opportunity their encounters opening up to others have not been awesome, and as a matter of fact, frequently were horrendous. In all probability, they will definitely disapprove of confidence in more ways than one. Regardless of where you land as far as trust, there are a lot of ways of developing your weakness and confidence in others.

It's essential to take note that trust issues in connections can frequently come from the two sides. As a matter of fact, the individual in recuperation might think their accomplice is cheating or lying, which might come from their own mental self-portrait challenges or in considering themselves to genuinely deserve their relationship. Essentially, an individual dating a recuperating alcoholic or somebody in recuperation can think their accomplice might have backslid or lied about different things. Open, legitimate correspondence is the best way to chip away at trust issues.

Be careful of the Gamble of Backslide

Dating a recuperating alcoholic or somebody in recuperation should incorporate the mindfulness required to think about high-risk circumstances. Being genuinely unpredictable and in progress leaves somebody in recuperation extraordinarily defenceless against this. Everybody associated with the relationship should know about these triggers.

On the off chance that you are dating a recuperating alcoholic or somebody in recuperation, you and their support ought to be their most memorable protection line with respect to backslide. Satisfying this job requires additional tender loving care and profound information on your accomplices' triggers, and the capacity to assist them with bypassing issues. In the event that you decide to date somebody in recuperation, you should teach yourself about endlessly backslide triggers. Then, at that point, carve out an opportunity to completely investigate what is happening and the relationship to track down ways of dominating to forestall a slip.

The significant thing isn't to permit minor circumstances to pass without managing them. The feeling of dread toward your accomplice backsliding shouldn't keep you away from imparting and adapting to triggers. Be mindful so as not to empower undesirable ways of behaving simply because you would rather not trigger them.

Right now is an ideal opportunity to recollect that caring for somebody in recuperation implies maintaining that they should succeed, and that must be a higher priority than the progress of the relationship. Having collectedness as the need will realign backslide counteraction procedures all through the recuperation interaction.

Know about Co-dependency

In recuperation, we frequently gloat about how irreplaceable a help group is to an effective recuperation. Your help group can be what saves your life — you're depending on them. The fact that co-dependency examples might arise makes it exactly when a heartfelt connection is likewise sprouting during recuperation, it is conceivable. In this manner, moving extraordinary feelings without accomplishing the internal work initially can be the destruction of both the relationship and collectedness.

Indications of co-dependency include:

Trouble with:

Settling on choices in a relationship

Distinguishing your sentiments

Conveying in a relationship

Esteeming the endorsement of others more than self-endorsement

Lacking confidence in self and having unfortunate confidence

Communicating separation anxieties or an over-the-top requirement for endorsement

Cherishing somebody in recuperation will require keeping sound limits around reliance and backing. These lines are frequently crossed by those with past close-to-home injuries and past addictions, making such connections progressively defenceless to co-dependency.

On the off chance that you are dating a recuperating alcoholic or another person in recuperation, recollect you are similarly as engaged with their collectedness as they are. On the off chance that you love somebody in recuperation, you have a ton of familiarity with close-to-home speculation.

Along these lines, it is additionally basic to know about your own psychological well-being status. Carving out an opportunity to consider yourself will keep you from collapsing under the heaviness of a committed relationship. To appropriately uphold an accomplice in recuperation, you should be solid as well.

Chapter 6

10 sober exercises for enslavement recuperation

Sober living isn't simple 100% of the time. It very well may be challenging to progress from a way of life of abusing medications and liquor to finish forbearance in the wake of finishing an enslavement treatment program. At the point when you enter recuperation, you really want structure, standard, positive help, and even things, for example, sober exercises to participate in which have not been all a piece of your past life.

Why Finding Sober Exercises Are Significant

Early recuperation can cause you to feel like you are on an out-of-control thrill ride of feelings. Weariness and available energy can be hazardous during this time when you might feel overpowered by fanatical considerations, triggers, and desires. Sober exercises can assist you with exploring enslavement recuperation. They comprise individual or gathering exercises that occupy you from recuperation stressors and at the same time offer the help you really want to remain sober.

Sober exercises are things you do or take part in that offer you some award. In recuperation, the award is forestalling backslide. Sober exercises accomplish more than forestall backslides, be that as it may. They can assist you with gaining some new useful knowledge, lead to better well-being, and encourage you. They could actually give you that thrill you want.

Ten sober exercises for enslavement recuperation.

1. Get more familiar with Enslavement

Information is power. It's difficult to battle something when you don't know anything about it. Finding out about the infection of enslavement gives you an understanding of your cerebrum and how it responds to medications or liquor. You likewise gain proficiency with the various gambling factors that place you in danger of fostering a substance use jumble. Knowing this assists you with supplanting risk factors with defensive factors that assist you with forestalling backslides.

2. Reward Your People Group

You presumably won't want to chip in or reward your local area in early recuperation. At any rate, do it. Reports from Harvard demonstrate chipping in is connected to positive physical and psychological well-being. It causes you to feel socially associated and facilitates discouragement and forlornness. It additionally brings down pressure and further develops circulatory strain, among other medical advantages. On the off chance that you love creatures, volunteer at a creature salvage.

3. Practice an Expertise

You have likely contemplated mastering another expertise or working on an ability. Whether figuring out how to play an instrument, cooking or baking, painting, composing, building, or learning another dialect, right now is an ideal opportunity to make it happen. Mastering another expertise incorporates further developing cerebrum science, diverting you from triggers and desires, and battling weariness.

4. Go to a Level-headed Occasion

Occasions happen each day that don't include the abuse of medications or liquor. Games, shows, dramatic plays, motion pictures, and sober care groups are only a couple of models. Ask a level-headed companion or individual care group part to go to an occasion with you. On the off chance that you live in a space with less movement, take a stab at beginning something of your own.

5. Begin Something Positive

Since it isn't accessible now doesn't mean it can't work out. On the off chance that you can't find the right care group that tends to every one of your requirements, begin one with someone else in recuperation. On the off chance that you can't find an activity gathering to join, make one. While beginning a genuinely new thing, don't attempt to do it single-handedly. Structure a board of trustees in which everybody assumes a part as opposed to everything falling onto your shoulders. Feeling overpowered can be a trigger.

6. Unwind

Recuperation can be distressing. You are relearning how to do everything without the guidance of substances. Furthermore, you experience day-to-day sets off that entice you to backslide. An excessive amount of pressure can adversely influence your psychological and actual well-being and endanger your collectedness. Contemplation, yoga, profound breathing, rest cleanliness, and figuring out how to relinquish the things beyond your control support unwinding and stress the executives.

7. View as Your Otherworldly Side

There are explanation programs that urge individuals to construct a relationship with a Higher Power. You can communicate your otherworldly associations in the manner that suits you best. The key is to find the advantages otherworldliness offers, similar to absolution of yourself as well as other people, tolerating liability, being considered responsible, showing appreciation, and tracking down your motivation.

8. Track down an Open Air Experience

Getting outside and taking part in exercises can support your state of mind, ease discouragement and decrease nervousness. At the point when you are outside, your body is moving and getting exercise, regardless of whether it isn't exhausting. You additionally take in vitamin D and supplements from the sun. This large number of results lower pressure.

9. Snicker

Snickering is an interaction that includes different cerebrum regions, including feelings that permit you to get a joke and think that it is entertaining. The cerebrum additionally utilizes comprehension to deal with something entertaining, setting off muscles that make you grin. Chuckling supports the state of mind and deliveries muscle pressure. It additionally diminishes pressure by bringing down chemicals like cortisol.

10. Spend time with Loved ones

You don't necessarily in every case must be participated in a movement or go to an occasion to keep up with collectedness. Some of the time, you simply need the help of loved ones who love you and need to assist you with forestalling backslide. Being more friendly with friends and family empowers you to reconnect and reconstruct your connections that were harmed by the abuse of liquor or medications.

Conclusion

Enslavement recuperation is a long-lasting interaction. Try not to attempt to rush it. All things being equal, consolidate exercises to fabricate a level-headed way of life that will endure. Here are a few last tips for enslavement recuperation:

On the off chance that you goof, look for treatment promptly to refocus.

Try not to thrash yourself sincerely on the off chance that you slip. It happens to a great many people. The key is to refocus.

Be straightforward with yourself. On the off chance that you are contemplating backsliding, speak the truth about it. Connect with somebody who comprehends and can assist you with managing your contemplations and desires.

Extend your encouraging group of people. The more level-headed individuals you stick around the better your possibilities of staying away from backsliding. In the event that you decide to stick around individuals with a functioning substance use jumble, your possibilities of backsliding are higher.

Keep a recuperation mentality. Your considerations impact your activities. On the off chance that you continually figure you will backslide, you will probably backslide. On the off chance that you figure you will remain sober, you will.

Focus on your recuperation. Join advocates, peers, companions, family, and others in sober exercises for enslavement recuperation. You can track down ways of accomplishing long-haul collectedness.

On the off chance that you battle with enslavement, you realize how disconnecting and frightening it very well may be. Enslavement influences each aspect of your life, and when you come to depend on medications or liquor, it can feel like you're failing to keep a grip on the things that make the biggest difference.

Fortunately, enslavement is treatable. A greater part of junkies never seeks proficient treatment, however, the individuals who really do go through treatment frequently have great results. What's more, in opposition to mainstream thinking, enslavement treatment isn't simply level-headed living and long stretches of thoughtless treatment meetings.

Today, numerous enslavement treatments are imaginative and non-traditional. Increasingly more treatment communities, including Characterizing Wellbeing, are zeroing in on experiential treatment as a method for assisting clients with building new abilities and conquer one of the kind difficulties.

There is a lot of proof to help the way that experiential treatments, particularly experience-based treatments, can make all the difference for the psyche, body, and soul. During recuperation, setting out on new undertakings can show recuperating junkies a great deal about themselves and their feelings.

Why You Ought to Take part in Undertakings During Recuperation

At the point when you're effectively manhandling medications or liquor, zeroing in on the things that make you a superior person is troublesome. Your substance misuse administers your life and directs everything you might do. On the off chance that you're at present seeking treatment for enslavement, or are in any event, taking into account it, you've made a significant initial phase in your excursion to collectedness.

Many individuals view recuperation as absolutely getting level-headed. Be that as it may, as a general rule, recuperation allows you a second opportunity in life. It offers you a chance to carry on with a better, more joyful, and seriously satisfying life. That is the reason recuperation is the ideal opportunity to attempt new things and go on a couple of undertakings in the meantime.

Contemplate the keep-going time you went on a genuine experience. It could have been quite a while back during your experience growing up, or simply last week. In any case, paying little mind to when it worked out, you most likely recollect how you felt at that time. Perhaps you felt a feeling of achievement in the wake of climbing to the highest point of a mountain, or you felt certain when you finished a difficult ropes course.

Any experience or new experience you have helps develop you personally. It expands your certainty, supports your confidence, and gives you a characteristic dopamine help.

Experience treatment gives a psychological and actual rush that is a lot better option in contrast to drinking or utilizing drugs. That is the reason many individuals get new side interests during recuperation that give them a "characteristic high."

After you go on an undertaking, you can think back and value how far you've come. Perhaps it was whenever you've first at any point genuinely ventured beyond your usual range of familiarity. It doesn't make any difference what issues you're battling with, or how old you are. Participating in experience treatment is a demonstrated method for supporting your psychological well-being, decreasing pressure, and fostering critical thinking techniques that you can use in reality.

What Advantages of Experience Treatment?

You could imagine that the main individuals who benefit from experience treatment are regular conceived experience searchers. Be that as it may, everybody can profit from experiencing treatment somehow. Indeed, even the shyest and most reluctant individuals can track down satisfaction in a thrilling experience.

During another experience or a major experience, individuals who experience the ill effects of injury frequently encounter their greatest feelings of trepidation and close-to-home road obstructions. At the point when another circumstance tests their psychological or actual strength, their prompt response may be to lose confidence in their capacity or work themselves out of it.

At the point when an individual leaves their usual range of familiarity, they are compelled to settle on a decision — either push through or surrender. During experience treatment, a client's instructors and companions are there to urge them to continue onward during testing times. Subsequently, the individual turns out to be intellectually more grounded and more enabled. They demonstrate to themselves that they are equipped for anything.

The illustrations got the hang of during an undertaking and continue into regular day-to-day existence. Individuals get the certainty to understand that they can conquer their enslavement. It shows them that they have the right stuff to change their mentality under tension. Enslavement recuperation begins with psychological well-being, and experience treatment tends to a significant number of the psychological obstructions that individuals face making a course for collectedness.